T0233604

SCID-5-AMPD

STRUCTURED CLINICAL INTERVIEW FOR THE
DSM-5® ALTERNATIVE MODEL FOR PERSONALITY DISORDERS

MODULE III

Structured Clinical Interview for
PERSONALITY DISORDERS
(INCLUDING PERSONALITY DISORDER–TRAIT SPECIFIED)

Michael B. First, M.D. • Andrew E. Skodol, M.D.
Donna S. Bender, Ph.D. • John M. Oldham, M.D.

Interviewee/ID#: _____   Interview date: _____ _____ _____
                                                              month   day   year

Clinician: _____

SCID-5-AMPD

STRUCTURED CLINICAL INTERVIEW FOR THE DSM-5®
ALTERNATIVE MODEL FOR PERSONALITY DISORDERS

MODULE III

STRUCTURED CLINICAL INTERVIEW FOR
PERSONALITY DISORDERS
(INCLUDING PERSONALITY DISORDER–TRAIT SPECIFIED)

Michael B. First, M.D.
Professor of Clinical Psychiatry, Columbia University College of Physicians and
Surgeons, and Research Psychiatrist, Division of Clinical Phenomenology,
New York State Psychiatric Institute, New York, New York

Andrew E. Skodol, M.D.
Research Professor of Psychiatry, University of Arizona College of Medicine,
Tucson, Arizona; and Adjunct Professor of Psychiatry, Columbia University College of
Physicians and Surgeons, New York, New York

Donna S. Bender, Ph.D.
Director, Counseling and Psychological Services, and
Clinical Professor of Psychiatry and Behavioral Sciences,
Tulane University, New Orleans, Louisiana

John M. Oldham, M.D.
Professor of Psychiatry,
Barbara and Corbin Robertson Jr. Endowed Chair for Personality Disorders,
Baylor College of Medicine, Houston, Texas

An overview of the Module III rationale, structure, and approach is presented in the
User's Guide for the SCID-5-AMPD. Please refer to that manual for proper procedure
for conducting the assessment.

Contents

Abbreviations

ASPD = Antisocial Personality Disorder; AVPD = Avoidant Personality Disorder; BPD = Borderline Personality Disorder; NPD = Narcissistic Personality Disorder; OCPD = Obsessive-Compulsive Personality Disorder; PD = Personality Disorder; PD-TS = Personality Disorder–Trait Specified; STPD= Schizotypal Personality Disorder.

GENERAL OVERVIEW FOR THE SCID-5-AMPD

I'm going to start by asking you some questions about yourself and about problems or difficulties you may have had. I'll be making some notes as we go along. Do you have any questions before we begin?

NOTE: Any current suicidal thoughts, plans, or actions should be thoroughly assessed by the clinician and action taken if necessary.

DEMOGRAPHIC DATA

How old are you?

GENDER: ___ Male ___ Female ___ Other (e.g., transgender)

Are you married?

> *IF YES:* **How long have you been married?**

> *IF NO:* **Do you have a partner?**

>> *IF YES:* **How long have you been together? Do you live with your partner? Have you ever been married?**

>> *IF NO:* **Have you ever been married?**

IF EVER MARRIED: **How many times have you been married?**

Do you have any children?

   IF YES: **How many? (What are their ages?)**

With whom do you live? (How many children under the age of 18 live in your household?)

EDUCATION AND WORK HISTORY

How far did you go in school*?*

IF FAILED TO COMPLETE A PROGRAM IN WHICH INDIVIDUAL WAS ENROLLED:
Why did you leave?

What kind of work do you do? (Do you work outside of your home?)

Have you always done that kind of work?

   IF NO: **What other kind of work have you done in the past?**

What's the longest you've worked at one place?

(continued on next page)

EDUCATION AND WORK HISTORY (*continued*)

Are you currently employed (getting paid)?

IF NO: **Why not?**

IF UNKNOWN: **Has there ever been a period of time when you were unable to work or go to school?**

IF YES: **Why was that?**

Have you ever been arrested, involved in a lawsuit, or had other legal trouble?

CURRENT AND PAST PERIODS OF PSYCHOPATHOLOGY

Have you ever seen anybody for emotional or psychiatric problems?

→ *IF YES:* **What was that for? (What treatment did you get? Any medications? When was that? When was the first time you ever saw someone for emotional or psychiatric problems?)**

→ *IF NO:* **Was there ever a time when you, or someone else, thought you should see someone because of the way you were feeling or acting? (Tell me more.)**

Have you ever seen anybody for problems with alcohol or drugs?

IF YES: **What was that for? (What treatment[s] did you get? Any medications? When was that?)**

Have you ever attended a self-help group, like Alcoholics Anonymous, Gamblers Anonymous, or Overeaters Anonymous?

IF YES: **What was that for? When was that?**

Thinking back over your whole life, have there been times when things were not going well for you or when you were emotionally upset? (Tell me about that. When was that? What was that like? What was going on? How were you feeling?)

Begin Module III with the following questions to get a basic sense of the interviewee's view of self, basic approach to life, and quality of interpersonal relationships.

PRELIMINARY QUESTIONS ABOUT VIEW OF SELF
AND QUALITY OF INTERPERSONAL RELATIONSHIPS

IF THE QUESTIONS BELOW HAVE ALREADY BEEN ASKED IN THE CONTEXT OF ADMINISTERING MODULE I OR MODULE II, SKIP THIS SECTION AND CONTINUE WITH **PART I: ASSESSMENT AND SCORING OF PERSONALITY DISORDER CRITERIA**, *PAGE 5.*

The purpose of this interview is to explore different ways in which you see yourself, your basic approach to life, and how you interact with other people. Let's start with some general questions about how you are as a person:

1.   **How would you describe yourself as a person?**

2.   **How do you think other people describe you?**

3.   **How do you generally feel about yourself?**

(continued on next page)

4.　　　**How successful would you say you are at getting the things you want in life? (Like having a satisfying relationship, a fulfilling career, close friends?)**

5.　　　**What are your relationships with other people like?**

6.　　　**Who are the most important people in your life? How do you get along with them?**

7.　　　**How well do you think you understand yourself?**

8.　　　**How well do you understand other people?**

PART I: ASSESSMENT AND SCORING OF PERSONALITY DISORDER CRITERIA

Interviewer Instructions

Assessment of Criterion A: Domains of Personality Functioning

Criterion A for the six specific personality disorders in the Alternative Model consists of characteristic difficulties in **four areas of personality functioning (self and interpersonal)**: Identity, Self-Direction, Empathy, and Intimacy. Each element is rated on a three-point scale: 0 = "Absent"; 1 = "Present but subthreshold" (i.e., not clinically significant); and 2 = "Present at threshold" (i.e., clinically significant). A rating of "?" indicates insufficient information to make a judgment about an area of functioning. *Clinical significance* is based on the amount of distress or impairment in self and interpersonal functioning that can be ascribed to each Criterion A manifestation. Mild distress or impairment would warrant a rating of "1"; moderate or greater impairment would warrant a rating of "2."

Ask all of the questions for each area of personality functioning and then make a single, overall rating of the degree to which impairment is present in that area for the interviewee. For each question, ask for examples and elaboration until you have sufficient information to make a judgment. It is important to keep in mind that many individuals lack extensive, if any, insight regarding their personality functioning. Thus, negative answers to questions should not necessarily be construed as sufficient evidence for deciding that a rating of "2" is not warranted.

The manifestations should be currently present and characterize the interviewee's personality functioning, in general, for at least the past 2 years. At least two of the four domains of the Criterion A for a given personality disorder must be rated "2" in order for Criterion A for that personality disorder to be met.

Assessment of Criterion B: Specific Trait Facets

Criterion B for the personality disorders in the Alternative Model specifies **a required number and, in some cases, pattern of personality trait facets.** Ask all of the questions for each facet and then make a single, overall rating of the degree to which each facet describes the interviewee. For each question, ask for examples and elaboration until you have sufficient information to make a judgment. You should ensure that elicited examples represent actual traits (i.e., general predispositions or tendencies) as opposed to more limited instances of behavior.

Personality facets within each domain are rated on a four-point scale of descriptiveness: 0 = "Very little or not at all descriptive," 1 = "Mildly descriptive," 2 = "Moderately descriptive," 3 = "Very descriptive." For a trait facet to be considered present and consequently count toward meeting Criterion B, a rating of "2" ("Moderately descriptive") or "3" ("Very descriptive") is required. The facets should describe the interviewee's current personality and be descriptive for at least the past 2 years. The facet descriptions usually contain multiple components. A rating of "3" does not necessarily require that all of the components are descriptive of the individual. If some subset of components is particularly descriptive, a rating of "3" may still be appropriate. A rating of "?" indicates that there is insufficient information to make a judgment about the descriptiveness of the facet.

(continued on next page)

For several trait facets, the general definition of the trait (from DSM-5, pp. 779–781) has been modified to better suit the personality disorder to which it applies, as in the Alternative Model. Because of these disorder-specific differences in trait definitions, there are disorder-specific differences in the interview questions.

Moreover, a number of traits appear in the criteria for two disorders. In order to avoid the interview being repetitive, the first time the trait is encountered in the interview, the interviewer asks the interviewee the questions for that trait and then applies the elicited response to the other disorder in which that trait appears. For some disorders, the wording of the trait definition is identical across disorders and thus the rating can be transcribed to whichever disorders it applies. For other disorders, the wording of the trait definition differs between the disorders and thus additional questions are given to facilitate the disorder-specific evaluation of that trait.

Making a Provisional Diagnosis, Then Evaluating Criteria C–G

At the end of each Criterion A section, the interviewer makes note of whether or not that Criterion A is met. At the end of each Criterion B section for each personality disorder, the interviewer makes note of whether or not that Criterion B is met. If both Criteria A and B are met for the specific personality disorder, a provisional diagnosis of the disorder is made. A definite diagnosis can be made only after determining whether Criteria C–G from the General Criteria for Personality Disorders have been met.

The interviewer should then refer to "Assessing Criteria C–G of General Criteria for Personality Disorder" (pages 48–49) whenever making that determination. This section is provided at the end of Part I (i.e., after the Personality Disorder Summary) for ease of reference. After Criteria C–G are evaluated for that particular disorder and the result is marked at the conclusion of Criterion B for that disorder, the interviewer returns to continue assessing each subsequent personality disorder in Part I.

Assessment of Personality Trait Facets Not Associated With Any Specific Personality Disorder

After the assessment of the diagnostic criteria for each of the six personality disorders, Part I continues with the assessment of personality trait facets not associated with any specific personality disorder; this component is included to cover all the personality trait facets presented in the Alternative Model and for the interviewer's use in evaluating PD-TS in Part II.

Personality Disorder Summary

Part I concludes with the Personality Disorder Summary, in which the interviewer notes the presence or absence of the six Alternative Model personality disorders. If criteria are met for at least one personality disorder, the interviewer continues with Part III: Rating Severity of the Personality Disorder: Level of Personality Functioning Scale. Otherwise, the interviewer continues with Part II: Evaluation of Personality Disorder—Trait Specified.

Note that at this point in the SCID-5-AMPD, all of the interview questions will have been asked (i.e., there are no additional interview questions in Parts II and III). The interviewer should conclude the interview and excuse the interviewee before completing Parts II and III.

Refer to the *User's Guide for the SCID-5-AMPD* for complete instructions on use of Module III.

Avoidant Personality Disorder

CRITERION A. Moderate or greater impairment in personality functioning, manifested by characteristic difficulties in two or more of the following four areas:

Interview questions	Criterion A definitions	Rating
Do you often feel that other people are judging you negatively in some way? Do you feel inept, unappealing, or inferior around other people? Do you often feel very ashamed? Do you believe that you're not as good, as smart, or as attractive as most other people?	1. **Identity:** Low self-esteem associated with self-appraisal as socially inept, personally unappealing, or inferior; excessive feelings of shame.	? 0 1 2
Are you so afraid to fail that you are reluctant to try to get what you want in life? Are you generally afraid to take risks in life? Are you afraid to try new things if they involve having to deal with other people? *IF YES TO ANY OF ABOVE:* **Is that because you tend to expect too much of yourself?**	2. **Self-Direction:** Unrealistic standards for behavior associated with reluctance to pursue goals, take personal risks, or engage in new activities involving interpersonal contact.	? 0 1 2

?	0	1	2
Insufficient information	Absent	Present but subthreshold	Present at threshold

Interview questions	Criterion A definitions	Rating
Are you frequently worried about being criticized by others? **Are you easily hurt by criticism or rejection?** **Are you often concerned that other people feel negatively about you?**	3. **Empathy:** Preoccupation with, and sensitivity to, criticism or rejection, associated with distorted inference of others' perspectives as negative.	? 0 1 2
Do you avoid getting involved with people unless you are certain they will like you? **Are you afraid to get close to another person because you worry that he or she might make you feel ashamed or ridicule you?** **When you are in a close relationship, do you still find it hard to share your thoughts and feelings?**	4. **Intimacy:** Reluctance to get involved with people unless being certain of being liked; diminished mutuality within intimate relationships because of fear of being shamed or ridiculed.	? 0 1 2
	At least <u>TWO</u> CRITERION A items are rated "2."	NO YES

Avoidant PD
Criterion A is met.

?	0	1	?
Insufficient information	**Absent**	**Present but subthreshold**	**Present at threshold**

CRITERION B. Three or more of the following four pathological personality traits, one of which must be (1) Anxiousness:

Interview questions	Criterion B definitions	Rating
	1. **Anxiousness** (an aspect of Negative Affectivity) *NOTE: This facet is included in both Avoidant PD and Borderline PD.*	**Avoidant PD (Criterion B1):** ? 0 1 2 3
FOR AVOIDANT PD (CRITERION B1): **Do you generally feel very nervous, anxious, or even panicky in social situations?**	(For **Avoidant PD:** Intense feelings of nervousness, tenseness, or panic, often in reaction to social situations;)	
		Borderline PD (Criterion B2):
FOR BORDERLINE PD (CRITERION B2): **How about feeling nervous, tense, or panicky when you are having a difficult time with a family member, friend, or romantic partner?**	(For **Borderline PD:** Intense feelings of nervousness, tenseness, or panic, often in reaction to interpersonal stresses;)	? 0 1 2 3
Are you almost always worrying about something?	Worry about the negative effects of past unpleasant experiences and future negative possibilities;	
Do you tend to dwell on the bad things that have happened to you in the past?		
What about worrying about bad things that might happen to you in the future?		
Do you tend to feel upset when things are up in the air or when you are uncertain about how things will turn out?	Feeling fearful, apprehensive, or threatened by uncertainty;	
Do situations like this, that is, when things are uncertain, make you feel threatened?		
	(continued on next page)	

?	0	1	2	3
Insufficient information	Very little or not at all descriptive	Mildly descriptive	Moderately descriptive	Very descriptive

Interview questions	Criterion B definitions	Rating
	1. **Anxiousness** (*continued*)	
FOR AVOIDANT PD (CRITERION B1): **Do you often worry about being embarrassed by the things you say or do?**	(For **Avoidant PD:** Fears of embarrassment.)	
FOR BORDERLINE PD (CRITERION B2): **How about often being afraid that at any moment you might fall apart or lose control?**	(For **Borderline PD:** Fears of falling apart or losing control.)	
	2. **Withdrawal** (an aspect of Detachment) *NOTE: This facet is included in both Avoidant PD and Schizotypal PD.*	**Avoidant PD (Criterion B2):**
Are you usually quiet when you meet new people?	Reticence in social situations;	? 0 1 2 3
Do you generally try to avoid social events?	Avoidance of social contacts and activity;	**Schizotypal PD (Criterion B5):**
Do you usually avoid starting conversations with people you don't know very well?	Lack of initiation of social contact.	? 0 1 2 3
FOR SCHIZOTYPAL PD (CRITERION B5): **Would you almost always rather do things alone than with other people? Why is that?**	(For **Schizotypal PD:** Preference for being alone to being with others)	

?	0	1	2	3
Insufficient information	Very little or not at all descriptive	Mildly descriptive	Moderately descriptive	Very descriptive

Interview questions	Criterion B definitions	Rating
Are there really very few things that give you pleasure? Do you feel like you don't have enough energy to take advantage of what life has to offer? Do you find that you do not get as much pleasure out of things as others seem to? Do you find that nothing seems to interest you very much?	3. **Anhedonia** (an aspect of Detachment) Lack of enjoyment from, engagement in, or energy for life's experiences; Deficits in the capacity to feel pleasure or take interest in things.	? 0 1 2 3
IF UNKNOWN: **What's the most satisfying romantic or sexual relationship that you have had? Tell me about it.** *ASK THE FOLLOWING QUESTIONS ONLY IF UNCLEAR FROM RELATIONSHIP HISTORY:* **Do you tend to avoid getting close to people? Why is that?** **Do you tend to break off relationships or friendships if they start to get close?** **Have you generally avoided getting into emotionally intimate sexual relationships?**	4. **Intimacy Avoidance** (an aspect of Detachment) *NOTE: This facet is included in both Avoidant PD and OCPD.* Avoidance of close or romantic relationships, interpersonal attachments, and intimate sexual relationships.	**Avoidant PD (Criterion B4)/ OCPD (Criterion B3):** ? 0 1 2 3
	At least <u>THREE</u> CRITERION B AVOIDANT PD TRAITS are rated "2" or "3" and <u>ONE</u> of these must be CRITERION B1: ANXIOUSNESS.	NO YES

Avoidant PD Criterion B is met.

?	0	1	2	3
Insufficient information	**Very little or not at all descriptive**	**Mildly descriptive**	**Moderately descriptive**	**Very descriptive**

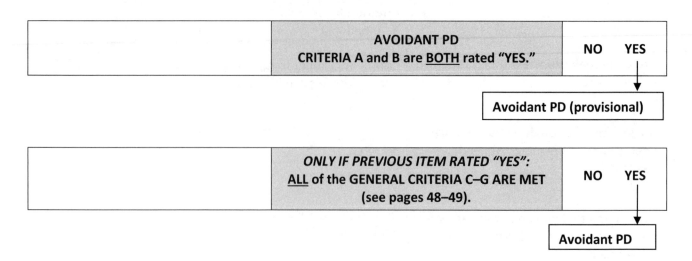

	AVOIDANT PD CRITERIA A and B are <u>BOTH</u> rated "YES."	NO YES

Avoidant PD (provisional)

	ONLY IF PREVIOUS ITEM RATED "YES": <u>ALL</u> of the GENERAL CRITERIA C–G ARE MET (see pages 48–49).	NO YES

Avoidant PD

?	0	1	2	3
Insufficient information	Very little or not at all descriptive	Mildly descriptive	Moderately descriptive	Very descriptive

Obsessive-Compulsive Personality Disorder

CRITERION A. Moderate or greater impairment in personality functioning, manifested by characteristic difficulties in two or more of the following four areas:

Interview questions	Criterion A definitions	Rating
Do you only feel good about yourself when you are working hard or accomplishing your goals? **Do you or other people feel that you are so devoted to work (or school) that you have no time left for anyone else or for just having fun?** **Do you get uncomfortable if you start experiencing strong emotions?** **Do you try not to show your emotions to other people?**	1. **Identity:** Sense of self derived predominantly from work or productivity; constricted experience and expression of strong emotions.	? 0 1 2

Are you a very careful person who likes to do things just right?
 	
Do you find it hard to finish tasks, jobs, or assignments?
 	
  IF YES: **Is this because you need everything to be perfect?**
 	
Are you a very moral person who strongly believes in "right" and "wrong"?
 	
  IF YES: **Do you think you have higher moral standards than most people?**
 	
Do you usually follow rules to the letter of the law, no matter what?
	2. **Self-Direction**: Difficulty completing tasks and realizing goals, associated with rigid and unreasonably high and inflexible internal standards of behavior; overly conscientious and moralistic attitudes.	? 0 1 2

?	0	1	2
Insufficient information	**Absent**	**Present but subthreshold**	**Present at threshold**

Interview questions	Criterion A definitions	Rating
Do you frequently wish you didn't have to bother trying to understand the ideas, feelings, and actions of others? **Do you believe so strongly in your ideals and values that you find it difficult to understand other people's points of view?**	3. **Empathy:** Difficulty understanding and appreciating the ideas, feelings, or behaviors of others.	? 0 1 2
Does it seem like you end up working so much that you hardly have any time left for relationships? **Do people seem to think you are stubborn or too invested in your way of doing things?** **Has the fact that you hold to your beliefs so strongly created problems in your relationships?**	4. **Intimacy:** Relationships seen as secondary to work and productivity; rigidity and stubbornness negatively affect relationships with others.	? 0 1 2
	At least <u>**TWO**</u> **CRITERION A items are rated "2."**	NO YES

Obsessive-Compulsive PD Criterion A is met.

?	0	1	2
Insufficient information	**Absent**	**Present but subthreshold**	**Present at threshold**

CRITERION B. Three or more of the following four pathological personality traits, one of which must be (1) Rigid Perfectionism:

Interview questions	Criterion B definitions	Rating
	1. **Rigid Perfectionism** (an aspect of extreme Conscientiousness, the opposite pole of Disinhibition)	? 0 1 2 3
Do you insist on perfection in everything you do? Tell me about that.	Rigid insistence on everything being flawless, perfect, and without errors or faults, including one's own and others' performance;	
Do you also insist that everything other people do be flawless and perfect?		
Do you have trouble finishing jobs because you spend so much time trying to get things exactly right?	Sacrificing of timeliness to ensure correctness in every detail;	
Do you tend to believe that in general, there is only one right way to do things?	Believing that there is only one right way to do things;	
Do you often end up doing things yourself to make sure they are done right?		
Once you have formed an opinion about something, do you rarely change your mind because you know you're right?	Difficulty changing ideas and/or viewpoint;	
Are you the kind of person who focuses on details, order, and organization or who likes to make lists and schedules? Give me some examples.	Preoccupation with details, organization, and order.	

?	0	1	2	3
Insufficient information	Very little or not at all descriptive	Mildly descriptive	Moderately descriptive	Very descriptive

Interview questions	Criterion B definitions	Rating
Do you tend to keep doing the same thing over and over again even though it is not getting you anywhere? **Do you tend to keep doing certain things the same way, even when it's clear that your approach is not working?**	2. **Perseveration** (an aspect of Negative Affectivity) Persistence at tasks long after the behavior has ceased to be functional or effective; Continuance of the same behavior despite repeated failures.	**? 0 1 2 3**
*This item was rated during assessment of Avoidant PD. REFER TO AVOIDANT PD CRITERION B4 ON **PAGE 11** and TRANSCRIBE RATING OF THE **OCPD**-SPECIFIC VERSION OF THIS TRAIT.*	3. **Intimacy Avoidance** (an aspect of Detachment) *NOTE: This facet is included in both Avoidant PD and OCPD.* Avoidance of close or romantic relationships, interpersonal attachments, and intimate sexual relationships.	**? 0 1 2 3**
Do you tend not to get emotional about things? **Do you find that books, movies, and music that other people find moving leave you cold?** **Do you find that nothing makes you very happy or very sad or very angry?** **Have people told you that it is difficult to know what you're feeling?**	4. **Restricted Affectivity** (an aspect of Detachment) *NOTE: This facet is included in both OCPD and Schizotypal PD.* Little reaction to emotionally arousing situations; Constricted emotional experience and expression; *(continued on next page)*	**OCPD (Criterion B4)/ Schizotypal PD (Criterion B4)** **? 0 1 2 3**

?	0	1	2	3
Insufficient information	Very little or not at all descriptive	Mildly descriptive	Moderately descriptive	Very descriptive

Interview questions	Criterion B definitions	Rating
Do you not seem to care about anything or anyone? *IF NO:* **Have other people complained that you are a cold person?**	4. **Restricted Affectivity** *(continued)* Indifference or coldness.	
	At least <u>THREE</u> CRITERION B OBSESSIVE-COMPULSIVE PD TRAITS are rated "2" or "3" and <u>ONE</u> of these must be CRITERION B1: RIGID PERFECTIONISM.	NO YES

Obsessive-Compulsive PD Criterion B is met.

	OBSESSIVE-COMPULSIVE PD CRITERIA A and B are <u>BOTH</u> rated "YES."	NO YES

Obsessive-Compulsive PD (provisional)

	ONLY IF PREVIOUS ITEM RATED "YES": <u>ALL</u> of the GENERAL CRITERIA C–G ARE MET (see pages 48–49).	NO YES

Obsessive-Compulsive PD

?	0	1	2	3
Insufficient information	**Very little or not at all descriptive**	**Mildly descriptive**	**Moderately descriptive**	**Very descriptive**

Narcissistic Personality Disorder

CRITERION A. Moderate or greater impairment in personality functioning, manifested by characteristic difficulties in two or more of the following four areas:

Interview questions	Criterion A definitions	Rating
Are you at your best mainly when other people are telling you how important you are or that what you've done is really special? **Do you feel bad about yourself if you don't get positive feedback on a regular basis?** **Do you feel upset or dejected when somebody fails to notice you or something you've done?** **Do people often fail to appreciate your very special talents or accomplishments?** **Have people told you that you have too high an opinion of yourself?**	1. **Identity**: Excessive reference to others for self-definition and self-esteem regulation; exaggerated self-appraisal (inflated or deflated, or vacillating between extremes); emotional regulation mirrors fluctuations in self-esteem.	? 0 1 2
Do you often decide what to do based on whether others will approve of you for it? **Could you be comfortable taking a job that wasn't impressive or high status?** **Do you think that it is inevitable that you will be successful?** **Do you think that success should come your way because you deserve it?**	2. **Self-Direction**: Goal setting based on gaining approval from others; personal standards unreasonably high in order to see oneself as exceptional, or too low based on a sense of entitlement; often unaware of own motivations. *(continued on next page)*	? 0 1 2

?	0	1	2
Insufficient information	**Absent**	**Present but subthreshold**	**Present at threshold**

Interview questions	Criterion A definitions	Rating
	2. **Self-Direction** *(continued)*	
Do you think that you don't need to try hard in order to be successful because things should come your way in any case?		
Do you find it hard to relate to the feelings and needs of others?	3. **Empathy**: Impaired ability to recognize or identify with the feelings and needs of others; excessively attuned to reactions of others, but only if perceived as relevant to self; over- or underestimation of own effect on others.	? 0 1 2
Are you not really interested in other people's problems or feelings?		
Have people complained to you that you don't listen to them or care about their feelings?		
Do you pay a lot of attention to how other people are reacting to you?		
How much impact do you think the way you feel or act has on other people?		
Have people told you that you don't seem to notice the impact of your behavior on them?		

?	0	1	2
Insufficient information	**Absent**	**Present but subthreshold**	**Present at threshold**

Interview questions	Criterion A definitions	Rating
Are the people in your life generally there mostly to make you feel good? Do you have a lot of people you call "friends" but with whom you do not feel very close? Is having a large number of friends important to you in order for you to feel good about yourself? When you are with your friends, do you find yourself spending much more time talking about what's going on in your life rather than on what's going on with them? Do you often find the details of your friends' lives somewhat boring? Have you made friends with people primarily because of their wealth, power, influence, or fame?	4. **Intimacy**: Relationships largely superficial and exist to serve self-esteem regulation; mutuality constrained by little genuine interest in others' experiences and predominance of a need for personal gain.	? 0 1 2
	At least <u>TWO</u> CRITERION A items are rated "2."	NO YES

Narcissistic PD
Criterion A is met.

?	0	1	2
Insufficient information	Absent	Present but subthreshold	Present at threshold

CRITERION B. Both of the following pathological personality traits:		
Interview questions	**Criterion B definitions**	**Rating**
	1. **Grandiosity** (an aspect of Antagonism)	? 0 1 2 3
Do you think it's not necessary to follow certain rules or social conventions when they get in the way?	Feelings of entitlement, either overt or covert;	
Do you feel that you are the kind of person who deserves special treatment?		
Have other people told you that you are self-centered and only talk about yourself?	Self-centeredness;	
Do you feel like you have unique qualities that few others possess?	Firmly holding to the belief that one is better than others;	
Do you feel like you're more important than most people?		
Do you often feel resentful that other people fail to appreciate your special qualities or abilities?		
Have people told you that you have too high an opinion of yourself?	Condescension toward others.	
Do you find that there are very few people who are worth your time and attention?		

?	0	1	2	3
Insufficient information	Very little or not at all descriptive	Mildly descriptive	Moderately descriptive	Very descriptive

Interview questions	Criterion B definitions	Rating
	2. **Attention Seeking** (an aspect of Antagonism)	**? 0 1 2 3**
Do you like to be the center of attention?	Excessive attempts to attract and be the focus of the attention of others;	
Do you try to draw attention to yourself by the way you act, dress, or look?		
Do you often do things in order to get others to admire you?	Admiration seeking.	
Do you like standing out in a crowd?		
	<u>BOTH</u> CRITERION B1 and CRITERION B2 NARCISSISTIC PD TRAITS are rated "2" or "3."	**NO YES**

→ **Narcissistic PD Criterion B is met.**

	NARCISSISTIC PD CRITERIA A and B are <u>BOTH</u> rated "YES."	**NO YES**

→ **Narcissistic PD (provisional)**

	ONLY IF PREVIOUS ITEM RATED "YES": **<u>ALL</u> of the GENERAL CRITERIA C–G ARE MET** **(see pages 48–49).**	**NO YES**

→ **Narcissistic PD**

?	0	1	2	3
Insufficient information	Very little or not at all descriptive	Mildly descriptive	Moderately descriptive	Very descriptive

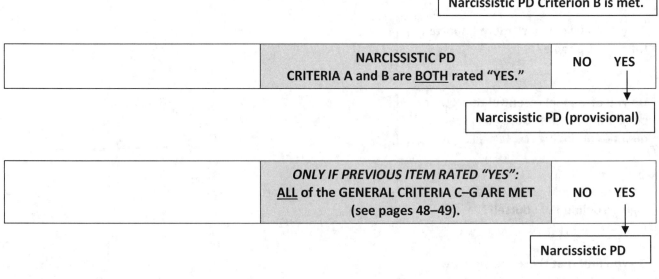

Borderline Personality Disorder

CRITERION A. Moderate or greater impairment in personality functioning, manifested by characteristic difficulties in two or more of the following four areas:

Interview questions	Criterion A definitions	Rating
Do you often have the sense that you don't know who you really are as a person? **Does your sense of yourself often change dramatically?** **Are you very self-critical and often feel like a bad person?** **Do you often feel empty inside?** **Do you "space out" when you feel very stressed?**	1. **Identity**: Markedly impoverished, poorly developed, or unstable self-image, often associated with excessive self-criticism; chronic feelings of emptiness; dissociative states under stress.	?　0　1　2
Do you often change your mind about what you want out of life? **Have you made many changes in where you went to school, your course of study, types of jobs you've had, or what you wanted to be?** **Have there been lots of sudden changes in your goals, values, career plans, religious beliefs, and so on?**	2. **Self-Direction**: Instability in goals, aspirations, values, or career plans.	?　0　1　2

?	0	1	2
Insufficient information	**Absent**	**Present but subthreshold**	**Present at threshold**

Interview questions	Criterion A definitions	Rating
Do you have trouble recognizing the feelings and needs of others? **Do you often feel slighted or insulted by others?** **Do you have trouble putting yourself in another person's shoes and seeing things through that person's eyes?** **Do you tend to focus on other people's flaws or weaknesses?**	3. **Empathy**: Compromised ability to recognize the feelings and needs of others associated with interpersonal hypersensitivity (i.e., prone to feel slighted or insulted); perceptions of others selectively biased toward negative attributes or vulnerabilities.	**? 0 1 2**
Do your relationships tend to be very intense? **Do your relationships with people you care about have a lot of ups and downs?** **When you are close to someone, is it difficult to trust that person?** **Do you often feel that your needs are not being met in your close relationships?** **Are you often worried that someone you are close to will leave you?** **Do you often put someone who is important to you on a pedestal, only to later find out that he or she didn't deserve it?**	4. **Intimacy**: Intense, unstable, and conflicted close relationships, marked by mistrust, neediness, and anxious preoccupation with real or imagined abandonment; close relationships often viewed in extremes of idealization and devaluation and alternating between over-involvement and withdrawal. *(continued on next page)*	**? 0 1 2**

?	0	1	2
Insufficient information	**Absent**	**Present but subthreshold**	**Present at threshold**

Interview questions	Criterion A definitions	Rating
Were there times when you thought your partner was everything you wanted and then other times when you thought he or she was a big disappointment? Do you sometimes tend to get too close to the important people in your life and at other times find it really hard to get close? Do you have periods in which you feel it is better to just keep to yourself?	4. **Intimacy** *(continued)*	
	At least <u>**TWO**</u> **CRITERION A items are rated "2."**	NO YES

Borderline PD
Criterion A is met.

?	0	1	2
Insufficient information	**Absent**	**Present but subthreshold**	**Present at threshold**

CRITERION B. Four or more of the following seven pathological personality traits, at least one of which must be (5) Impulsivity, (6) Risk Taking, or (7) Hostility:

Interview questions	Criterion B definitions	Rating
Would you consider yourself to be a very emotional person? *IF NO:* **Do other people consider you to be very moody?** **Do your emotions often change suddenly, quickly going from happy to angry or sad?** **Do you tend to react very strongly to things that happen to you?** *IF NO:* **Have people told you that your emotional reactions are more intense than they should be, given the circumstances?**	**1. Emotional Lability** (an aspect of Negative Affectivity) Unstable emotional experiences and frequent mood changes; Emotions that are easily aroused, intense, and/or out of proportion to events and circumstances.	? 0 1 2 3
*This item was rated during assessment of Avoidant PD. REFER TO AVOIDANT PD CRITERION B1 ON **PAGE 9** and TRANSCRIBE RATING OF THE **BORDERLINE PD**–SPECIFIC VERSION OF THIS TRAIT.*	**2. Anxiousness** (an aspect of Negative Affectivity) *NOTE: This facet is included in both Avoidant PD and Borderline PD.* Intense feelings of nervousness, tenseness, or panic, often in reaction to interpersonal stresses; Worry about the negative effects of past unpleasant experiences and future negative possibilities; Feeling fearful, apprehensive, or threatened by uncertainty; Fears of falling apart or losing control.	? 0 1 2 3

?	0	1	2	3
Insufficient information	**Very little or not at all descriptive**	**Mildly descriptive**	**Moderately descriptive**	**Very descriptive**

Interview questions	Criterion B definitions	Rating
	3. **Separation Insecurity** (an aspect of Negative Affectivity) Fears of rejection by—and/or separation from—significant others, associated with fears of excessive dependency and complete loss of autonomy.	? 0 1 2 3
Do you often worry that you will be rejected or abandoned by people you are involved with?		
Do you tend to get very anxious when you are separated from those you depend on?		
Do you worry a lot about being left alone to take care of yourself physically or emotionally?		
In relationships, do you go back and forth between feeling very clingy and dependent at some times and desperately needing your space at other times? Tell me about that.		
	4. **Depressivity** (an aspect of Negative Affectivity) Frequent feelings of being down, miserable, and/or hopeless;	? 0 1 2 3
Do you often feel down, depressed, or miserable?		
Does the future look really hopeless to you?		
Once you start feeling depressed, is it hard for you to snap out of it?	Difficulty recovering from such moods;	
Do you almost always expect things to turn out badly?	Pessimism about the future;	
	(continued on next page)	

?	0	1	2	3
Insufficient information	**Very little or not at all descriptive**	**Mildly descriptive**	**Moderately descriptive**	**Very descriptive**

Interview questions	Criterion B definitions	Rating
	4. **Depressivity** *(continued)*	
Do you feel ashamed about a lot of things? What about?	Pervasive shame;	
Do you believe that you are basically an inadequate person and often don't feel good about yourself?	Feelings of inferior self-worth;	
Do you often feel like a failure?		
Do you generally feel like the world would be better off if you were dead?	Thoughts of suicide and suicidal behavior.	
Have you sometimes had thoughts of killing yourself?		
Have you ever done anything to try to take your own life or made plans to do so?		

?	0	1	2	3
Insufficient information	Very little or not at all descriptive	Mildly descriptive	Moderately descriptive	Very descriptive

Interview questions	Criterion B definitions	Rating
	5. **Impulsivity** (an aspect of Disinhibition) *NOTE: This facet is included in both Borderline PD and Antisocial PD.*	**Borderline PD (Criterion B5):** **? 0 1 2 3**
Do you often do things on the spur of the moment without thinking about how it will affect you or other people?	Acting on the spur of the moment in response to immediate stimuli;	**Antisocial PD (Criterion B6):** **? 0 1 2 3**
When something happens to you, do you usually react immediately and without thinking about it? Tell me about that.		
Have you often done things impulsively, like buying things you really couldn't afford, having sex with people you hardly knew, having unsafe sex, or driving recklessly?		
Do you find that you often make rash decisions without adequately considering the possible outcomes?	Acting on a momentary basis without a plan or consideration of outcomes;	
Do you find it difficult to make plans or to stick with them?	Difficulty establishing or following plans;	
FOR BORDERLINE PD (Criterion B5): **When you are under a lot of stress, do you do things, such as cutting, burning, or scratching yourself?** *IF YES:* **Do you feel a sense of urgency to do these things?**	(For **Borderline PD**: A sense of urgency and self-harming behavior under emotional distress.)	

?	0	1	2	3
Insufficient information	**Very little or not at all descriptive**	**Mildly descriptive**	**Moderately descriptive**	**Very descriptive**

Interview questions	Criterion B definitions	Rating
Are you drawn to thrilling activities, even if they are very dangerous or risky? **Do you often engage in dangerous or risky activities regardless of your lack of training or experience?**	6. **Risk Taking** (an aspect of Disinhibition) *NOTE: This facet is included in both Borderline PD and Antisocial PD.* Engagement in dangerous, risky, and potentially self-damaging activities, unnecessarily and without regard to consequences;	**Borderline PD (Criterion B6)** ? 0 1 2 3 **Antisocial PD (Criterion B5):** ? 0 1 2 3
Would other people describe you as reckless? **Do you do a lot of things that others would consider risky?**	Lack of concern for one's limitations and denial of the reality of personal danger;	
FOR ANTISOCIAL PD (CRITERION B5): **Are you frequently bored?** *IF YES:* **When you're bored, do you feel driven to immediately do something to relieve that feeling?**	(For **Antisocial PD:** Boredom proneness and thoughtless initiation of activities to counter boredom.)	

?	0	1	2	3
Insufficient information	**Very little or not at all descriptive**	**Mildly descriptive**	**Moderately descriptive**	**Very descriptive**

Interview questions	Criterion B definitions	Rating
	7. **Hostility** (an aspect of Antagonism) *NOTE: This facet is included in both* *Borderline PD and Antisocial PD.*	**Borderline PD** **(Criterion B7)** **? 0 1 2 3**
Are you angry much of the time?	Persistent or frequent angry feelings;	
Are you easily angered?	Anger or irritability in response to minor slights and insults.	**Antisocial PD** **(Criterion B4):** **? 0 1 2 3**
Do you often get angry or lash out when someone criticizes or insults you in some way?		
Do you often snap at people when they do little things that irritate you?		
FOR ANTISOCIAL PD (CRITERION B4): **Do you feel it's very important to get back at people who have hurt you or done you wrong?**	(for **Antisocial PD**: Mean, nasty, or vengeful behavior.)	
FOR ANTISOCIAL PD (CRITERION B4): **Would you say that you have a mean or nasty streak?** *IF NO:* **Do others often accuse you of being mean or of doing nasty things to them?**		
	At least <u>FOUR</u> CRITERION B **BORDERLINE PD TRAITS** are rated "2" or "3" and at least <u>ONE</u> of these must be **CRITERION B5: IMPULSIVITY; CRITERION B6: RISK TAKING; or CRITERION B7: HOSTILITY.**	**NO YES** ↓

Borderline PD Criterion B is met.

?	0	1	2	3
Insufficient information	**Very little or not at all descriptive**	**Mildly descriptive**	**Moderately descriptive**	**Very descriptive**

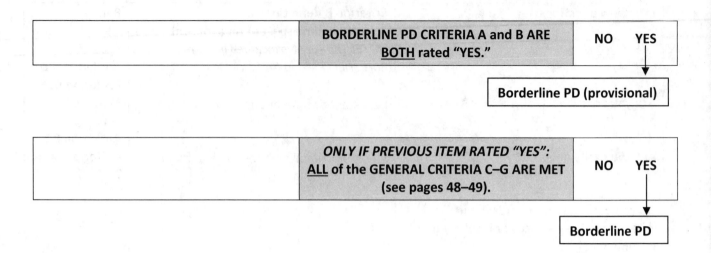

Antisocial Personality Disorder

CRITERION A. Moderate or greater impairment in personality functioning, manifested by characteristic difficulties in two or more of the following four areas:

Interview questions	Criterion A definitions	Rating
Is it really important to you to be in a position of power over others, to have others know you are the boss? **Do you only feel good about yourself when you have the upper hand?** **Are material possessions or a lot of wealth really important to how you see yourself?**	1. **Identity**: Egocentrism; self-esteem derived from personal gain, power, or pleasure.	**? 0 1 2**
Do you often try to get your needs met regardless of the consequences? **Have you done things that are against the law—even if you weren't caught— like stealing, using or selling drugs, writing bad checks, or having sex for money?** *IF NO:* **Have you ever been arrested for anything?**	2. **Self-Direction**: Goal setting based on personal gratification; absence of prosocial internal standards, associated with failure to conform to lawful or culturally normative ethical behavior.	**? 0 1 2**

? **Insufficient information**	**0** **Absent**	**1** **Present but subthreshold**	**2** **Present at threshold**

Interview questions	Criterion A definitions	Rating
How much does it bother you if you know that you have hurt or mistreated another person? Do you care about the feelings or needs of people other than yourself? Is it so important for you to get your needs met that others sometimes get hurt in the process? Have other people said that you have often used them to get what you want?	3. **Empathy:** Lack of concern for feelings, needs, or suffering of others; lack of remorse after hurting or mistreating another.	? 0 1 2
Do you often pretend to be in love with someone to get what you want, like sex? Do you only look for people who can help you get what you want? Do you think it is okay to lie to another person in order to get what you want? Do you find that you sometimes have to intimidate people to get your needs met? Do you often threaten other people to get what you want from them?	4. **Intimacy:** Incapacity for mutually intimate relationships, as exploitation is a primary means of relating to others, including by deceit and coercion; use of dominance or intimidation to control others.	? 0 1 2
	At least <u>TWO</u> CRITERION A items are rated "2."	NO YES

Antisocial PD
Criterion A is met.

?	0	1	2
Insufficient information	Absent	Present but subthreshold	Present at threshold

CRITERION B. Six or more of the following seven pathological personality traits:		
Interview questions	Criterion B definitions	Rating
Are you good at making other people do what you want them to?	1. **Manipulativeness** (an aspect of Antagonism) Frequent use of subterfuge to influence or control others;	? 0 1 2 3
Is it easy for you to take advantage of others?		
Do you bend the truth in order to get other people to do what you need them to do?		
Do you often "turn on the charm" or behave seductively in order to get what you want?	Use of seduction, charm, glibness, or ingratiation to achieve one's ends.	
Do you praise people when you don't mean it in order to get them to do what you want?		

?	0	1	2	3
Insufficient information	Very little or not at all descriptive	Mildly descriptive	Moderately descriptive	Very descriptive

Interview questions	Criterion B definitions	Rating
	2. **Callousness** (an aspect of Antagonism)	? 0 1 2 3
Do you tend to feel that other people's feelings or problems are not your concern?	Lack of concern for feelings or problems of others;	
Do you generally feel like it's no big deal if you hurt other people's feelings?		
If someone gets hurt because of something you do, do you feel guilty or sorry?	Lack of guilt or remorse about the negative or harmful effects of one's actions on others;	
Have you hit people or damaged property without really caring that you did so?	Aggression;	
Do you sometimes enjoy it when others are suffering or in pain?	Sadism.	

?	0	1	2	3
Insufficient information	Very little or not at all descriptive	Mildly descriptive	Moderately descriptive	Very descriptive

Interview questions	Criterion B definitions	Rating
Do you tend to exaggerate in order to get ahead? Do you often cheat in order to get what you want? Do you find that lying comes easily to you? Have you often "conned" others to get what you want? Have you ever used an "alias" or pretended you were somebody else? Do you tend to make things up when telling others about yourself? Do you often make up stories about things that happened that are totally untrue?	3. **Deceitfulness** (an aspect of Antagonism) Dishonesty and fraudulence; Misrepresentation of self; Embellishment or fabrication when relating events.	**? 0 1 2 3**
*This item was rated during assessment of Borderline PD. REFER TO BORDERLINE PD CRITERION B7 ON **PAGE 31** and TRANSCRIBE RATING OF THE **ANTISOCIAL PD**–SPECIFIC VERSION OF THIS TRAIT.*	4. **Hostility** (an aspect of Antagonism): Persistent or frequent angry feelings; anger or irritability in response to minor slights and insults; Mean, nasty, or vengeful behavior.	**? 0 1 2 3**

? **Insufficient information**	0 **Very little or not at all descriptive**	1 **Mildly descriptive**	2 **Moderately descriptive**	3 **Very descriptive**

Interview questions	Criterion B definitions	Rating
*This item was rated during assessment of Borderline PD. REFER TO BORDERLINE PD CRITERION B6 ON **PAGE 30** and TRANSCRIBE RATING OF THE **ANTISOCIAL PD**–SPECIFIC VERSION OF THIS TRAIT.*	5. **Risk Taking** (an aspect of Disinhibition): *NOTE: This facet is included in both Borderline PD and Antisocial PD.* Engagement in dangerous, risky, and potentially self-damaging activities, unnecessarily and without regard for consequences; Boredom proneness and thoughtless initiation of activities to counter boredom; Lack of concern for one's limitations and denial of the reality of personal danger.	? 0 1 2 3
*This item was rated during assessment of Borderline PD. REFER TO BORDERLINE PD CRITERION B5 ON **PAGE 29** and TRANSCRIBE RATING OF THE **ANTISOCIAL PD**–SPECIFIC VERSION OF THIS TRAIT.*	6. **Impulsivity** (an aspect of Disinhibition): *NOTE: This facet is included in both Borderline PD and Antisocial PD.* Acting on the spur of the moment in response to immediate stimuli; Acting on a momentary basis without a plan or consideration of outcomes; Difficulty establishing and following plans.	? 0 1 2 3
Have you ever owed people money and not paid them back? **What about not paying child support or not giving money to children or someone else who depended on you?** **Have you ever filed for bankruptcy? (How many times?)**	7. **Irresponsibility** (an aspect of Disinhibition) Disregard for—and failure to honor—financial and other obligations or commitments; *(continued on next page)*	? 0 1 2 3

?	0	1	2	3
Insufficient information	**Very little or not at all descriptive**	**Mildly descriptive**	**Moderately descriptive**	**Very descriptive**

Interview questions	Criterion B definitions	Rating
Do you tend to make promises that you don't keep? **Do you tend to skip important meetings and appointments if you don't feel like going?** **Do others consider you to be irresponsible?**	**7. Irresponsibility** *(continued)* Lack of respect for—and lack of follow-through on—agreements and promises.	

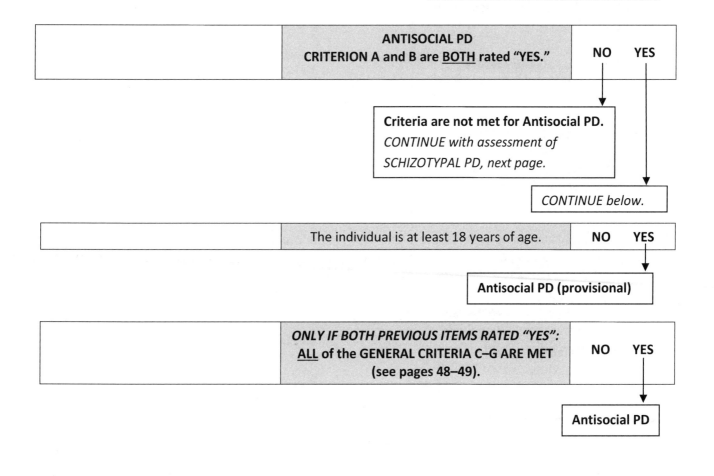

	At least <u>SIX</u> **CRITERION B** **ANTISOCIAL PD TRAITS are rated "2" OR "3."**	NO YES

Antisocial PD Criterion B is met.

	ANTISOCIAL PD **CRITERION A and B are <u>BOTH</u> rated "YES."**	NO YES

Criteria are not met for Antisocial PD. *CONTINUE with assessment of SCHIZOTYPAL PD, next page.*

CONTINUE below.

	The individual is at least 18 years of age.	NO YES

Antisocial PD (provisional)

	ONLY IF BOTH PREVIOUS ITEMS RATED "YES": <u>**ALL**</u> of the **GENERAL CRITERIA C–G ARE MET** (see pages 48–49).	NO YES

Antisocial PD

?	0	1	2	3
Insufficient information	**Very little or not at all descriptive**	**Mildly descriptive**	**Moderately descriptive**	**Very descriptive**

Schizotypal Personality Disorder

CRITERION A. Moderate or greater impairment in personality functioning, manifested by characteristic difficulties in two or more of the following four areas:

Interview questions	Criterion A definitions	Rating
Do you sometimes completely lose the sense of who you are when interacting with others? **Do you often take on the emotions and ideas of people you identify with?** **Does being around other people sometimes make you feel confused about who you really are?** **Are you very different from most people you know?** *IF YES*: **In what ways do you see yourself as different?** **Have other people told you that your emotions seem disconnected with what's going on, for example, laughing or acting silly when something really bad is happening?**	1. **Identity**: Confused boundaries between self and others; distorted self-concept; emotional expression often not congruent with context or internal experience.	? 0 1 2
Do you often feel like you have no idea of what you want out of life? **Have people told you that your goals in life are unrealistic because you don't have what's needed to accomplish them?** **Are you often confused about issues of "right" and "wrong"?**	2. **Self-Direction**: Unrealistic or incoherent goals; no clear set of internal standards.	? 0 1 2

?	0	1	2
Insufficient information	**Absent**	**Present but subthreshold**	**Present at threshold**

Interview questions	Criterion A definitions	Rating
Are you often confused about how your behavior appears to affect others? Do you often not understand why someone else is acting as he or she is toward you? Do other people's behavior or motivations seem mysterious to you most of the time?	3. **Empathy**: Pronounced difficulty understanding impact of own behaviors on others; frequent misinterpretations of others' motivations and behaviors.	? 0 1 2
Do you find it easier to relate to people online rather than in the real world? Is it hard for you to get close to people because you find it hard to trust them? Does being around other people cause you to feel a lot of anxiety?	4. **Intimacy**: Marked impairments in developing close relationships, associated with mistrust and anxiety.	? 0 1 2
	At least <u>TWO</u> CRITERION A items are rated "2."	NO YES

Schizotypal PD
Criterion A is met.

CRITERION B. Four or more of the following six pathological personality traits:		
Interview questions	**Criterion B definitions**	**Rating**
CONSIDER INTERVIEWEE'S SPEECH AND THINKING PROCESSES DURING THE INTERVIEW.	1. **Cognitive and Perceptual Dysregulation** (an aspect of Psychoticism)	? 0 1 2 3
Do your thoughts often go off in odd or unusual directions? *IF NO:* **Have others told you that your thoughts do not make sense to them?**	Odd or unusual thought processes;	
Do other people sometimes complain that when you speak, you veer off on tangents and have trouble getting to the point?	Vague, circumstantial, metaphorical, overelaborate, or stereotyped thought or speech;	
Do other people often tell you that you are too vague when expressing yourself?		
Do other people often tell you that you go into too much detail when recounting a story?		
Do you sometimes hear things that others couldn't hear?	Odd sensations in various sensory modalities.	
Do you see things that aren't actually there?		

?	0	1	2	3
Insufficient information	**Very little or not at all descriptive**	**Mildly descriptive**	**Moderately descriptive**	**Very descriptive**

Interview questions	Criterion B definitions	Rating
	2. **Unusual Beliefs and Experiences** (an aspect of Psychoticism)	? 0 1 2 3
Do you sometimes believe that you can read other people's minds?	Thought content and views of reality that are viewed by others as bizarre or idiosyncratic;	
How about being able to physically move things simply by thinking about moving them?		
Have you sometimes felt that you could make things happen or influence people just by making a wish or thinking about them?		
Do you believe that you have a "sixth sense" that allows you to know and predict things that others can't?		
Have you sometimes had the sense that some person or force is around you even though you cannot see anyone?	Unusual experiences of reality.	
Have you ever felt someone outside of yourself may be controlling your thoughts?		
Have you had personal experiences with the supernatural?		
Have you had weird experiences that are difficult to explain?		
Have you had any other experiences that you or someone else might consider unusual?		

?	0	1	2	3
Insufficient information	**Very little or not at all descriptive**	**Mildly descriptive**	**Moderately descriptive**	**Very descriptive**

Interview questions	Criterion B definitions	Rating
ALSO CONSIDER INTERVIEWEE'S APPEARANCE AND BEHAVIOR DURING THE INTERVIEW. **Do other people seem to think your behavior is odd, eccentric, or weird?** **Do others seem to think that you act, talk, or look odd, strange, or unusual?** **Have you been told that you have a number of odd quirks or habits?**	3. **Eccentricity** (an aspect of Psychoticism) Odd, unusual, or bizarre behavior or appearance; saying unusual or inappropriate things.	? 0 1 2 3
*This item was rated during assessment of OCPD. REFER TO OCPD CRITERION B4 ON **PAGE 16** and TRANSCRIBE RATING OF THE **SCHIZOTYPAL PD**–SPECIFIC VERSION OF THIS TRAIT.*	4. **Restricted Affectivity** (an aspect of Detachment) *NOTE: This facet is included in both OCPD and Schizotypal PD.* Little reaction to emotionally arousing situations; Constricted emotional experience and expression; Indifference or coldness.	? 0 1 2 3
*This item was rated during assessment of Avoidant PD. REFER TO AVOIDANT PD CRITERION B2 ON **PAGE 10** and TRANSCRIBE RATING OF THE **SCHIZOTYPAL PD**–SPECIFIC VERSION OF THIS TRAIT.*	5. **Withdrawal** (an aspect of Detachment) *NOTE: This facet is included in both Avoidant PD and Schizotypal PD.* Preference for being alone to being with others; Reticence in social situations; Avoidance of social contacts and activity; Lack of initiation of social contact.	? 0 1 2 3

?	0	1	2	3
Insufficient information	**Very little or not at all descriptive**	**Mildly descriptive**	**Moderately descriptive**	**Very descriptive**

Interview questions	Criterion B definitions	Rating
Do you often have to keep an eye out to stop people from using you or hurting you? **Are you especially sensitive to how other people treat you?** **Do you find that it is best not to let other people know much about you because they will use it against you?** **Do you spend a lot of time wondering if you can trust your friends or the people you work with?** **Have you often suspected that your spouse or partner has been unfaithful?** **Do you often feel like you are being harassed or treated cruelly or unfairly by others?**	6. **Suspiciousness** (an aspect of Detachment) Expectations of—and heightened sensitivity to—signs of interpersonal ill-intent or harm; Doubts about loyalty and fidelity of others; Feelings of persecution.	? 0 1 2 3
	At least <u>FOUR</u> CRITERION B SCHIZOTYPAL PD TRAITS are rated "2" or "3."	NO YES

Schizotypal PD Criterion B is met.

	SCHIZOTYPAL PD CRITERIA A and B are <u>BOTH</u> rated "YES."	NO YES

Schizotypal PD (provisional)

	***ONLY IF PREVIOUS ITEM RATED "YES":* ALL of the GENERAL CRITERIA C–G ARE MET** (see pages 48–49).	NO YES

Schizotypal PD

?	0	1	2	3
Insufficient information	**Very little or not at all descriptive**	**Mildly descriptive**	**Moderately descriptive**	**Very descriptive**

Personality Trait Facets Not Associated
With Any Specific Personality Disorder

Interview questions	Trait definitions	Rating
	Submissiveness (an aspect of Negative Affectivity) Adaptation of one's behavior to the actual or perceived interests and desires of others even when doing so is antithetical to one's own interests, needs, or desires.	? 0 1 2 3
Do you find it hard to disagree with people even when you think they are wrong?		
Do you tend to put other people's interests, needs, or desires before your own even when they go against your own?		
Do you always try to find out what other people want before deciding what you want for yourself?		
Do you usually do what you think others want you to do?		
	Distractibility (an aspect of Disinhibition) Difficulty concentrating and focusing on tasks; attention is easily diverted by extraneous stimuli;	? 0 1 2 3
Do you tend to find it hard to concentrate and focus on tasks?		
Do you tend to be easily distracted by things around you so that you have trouble concentrating or staying on one track?		
Do you have trouble pursuing specific goals, even for short periods of time?	Difficulty maintaining goal-focused behavior, including both planning and completing tasks.	
Do you have trouble planning and completing tasks?		

?	0	1	2	3
Insufficient information	Very little or not at all descriptive	Mildly descriptive	Moderately descriptive	Very descriptive

Personality Disorder Summary

Complete the table below to indicate the presence of one (or more) of the specific personality disorders (i.e., Criteria A through G are met).

Avoidant Personality Disorder (page 12)	**Absent**	**Present**
Obsessive-Compulsive Personality Disorder (page 17)	**Absent**	**Present**
Narcissistic Personality Disorder (page 22)	**Absent**	**Present**
Borderline Personality Disorder (page 32)	**Absent**	**Present**
Antisocial Personality Disorder (page 39)	**Absent**	**Present**
Schizotypal Personality Disorder (page 45)	**Absent**	**Present**

IF CRITERIA ARE <u>NOT</u> MET for AT LEAST ONE of the SIX SPECIFIC PERSONALITY DISORDERS, CONTINUE with PART II, "EVALUATION OF PERSONALITY DISORDER–TRAIT SPECIFIED," on page 50.

IF CRITERIA <u>ARE</u> MET for <u>AT LEAST ONE</u> of the SIX SPECIFIC PERSONALITY DISORDERS, CONTINUE with PART III, "RATING SEVERITY OF THE PERSONALITY DISORDER: LEVEL OF PERSONALITY FUNCTIONING SCALE," on page 53.

Assessing Criteria C–G
of General Criteria for Personality Disorder

Evaluate the following General Criteria for Personality Disorder when determining whether a particular personality disorder diagnosis can be made once it has been established that **Criterion A (impairments in personality functioning) and Criterion B (required pathological personality traits) have been met.**

Personality Disorder–Trait Specified is evaluated in Part II; refer back to this assessment when prompted there.

Interview questions	Criterion definitions	Criterion met? (for applicable PD)*
IF UNKNOWN: **Are** [THESE IMPAIRMENTS AND TRAITS] **present in a lot of different situations?** *IF UNKNOWN:* **Do** [THESE IMPAIRMENTS AND TRAITS] **occur with a lot of different people?**	**CRITERION C.** The impairments in personality functioning and the individual's personality trait expression are <u>relatively inflexible and pervasive</u> across a broad range of personal and social situations. *Note: A personality disorder item should be expressed consistently across most situations and not be restricted to a single interpersonal relationship, situation, or role.*	AVPD OCPD NPD BPD ASPD STPD PD-TS
IF UNKNOWN: **Have you been this way for a long time?** *IF UNKNOWN:* **How often does this happen?** *IF UNKNOWN:* **When can you first remember (feeling/acting/thinking) this way?**	**CRITERION D.** The impairments in personality functioning and the individual's personality trait expression are <u>relatively stable across time</u>, with onsets that can be traced back to at least adolescence or early adulthood. *Note: A personality disorder item must have been frequently present over a period of at least the last 2 years and there must be evidence of the characteristics going back as far as the late teens or early 20s.*	AVPD OCPD NPD BPD ASPD STPD PD-TS
IF THERE IS EVIDENCE OF ANOTHER MENTAL DISORDER WITH SYMPTOMS THAT RESEMBLE THE PERSONALITY ITEM IN QUESTION: **Does this happen only when you are having** [SXS OF MENTAL DISORDER]**?**	**CRITERION E.** The impairments in personality functioning and the individual's personality trait expression are <u>not better explained by another mental disorder</u>. *Note: If another mental disorder has been present, the course of the personality disorder must occur independently of the other mental disorder (e.g., onset prior to the other mental disorder or is significant when the other mental disorder is not prominent.)*	AVPD OCPD NPD BPD ASPD STPD PD-TS

Interview questions	Criterion definitions	Criterion met? (for applicable PD)*
IF THERE IS EVIDENCE OF PROLONGED EXCESSIVE ALCOHOL OR DRUG USE THAT RESULTS IN SYMPTOMS THAT RESEMBLE THE PERSONALITY ITEM IN QUESTION: **Does this happen only when you are drunk or high or withdrawing from alcohol or drugs?** **Does this happen only when you are trying to get alcohol or drugs?** *IF THERE IS EVIDENCE OF ANOTHER MEDICAL CONDITION THAT RESULTS IN SYMPTOMS THAT RESEMBLE THE PERSONALITY ITEM IN QUESTION:* **Were you like that before [ONSET OF ANOTHER MEDICAL CONDITION]?**	**CRITERION F.** The impairments in personality functioning and the individual's personality trait expression are <u>not solely attributable to the [direct] physiological effects of a substance or another medical condition</u> (e.g., severe head trauma). *Note: If there is a history of chronic substance use, the personality disorder is not better explained as a manifestation of chronic recurrent Substance Intoxication or Substance Withdrawal and is not exclusively associated with activities in the service of sustaining substance use (e.g., antisocial behavior). If another medical condition is present, the personality disorder manifestations are not better explained as a direct physiological consequence of the other medical condition.*	AVPD OCPD NPD BPD ASPD STPD PD-TS
ARE THE INDIVIDUAL'S IMPAIRMENTS AND TRAITS IN EXCESS OF WHAT MIGHT BE EXPECTED GIVEN THE INDIVIDUAL'S AGE AND CULTURAL CONTEXT?	**CRITERION G.** The impairments in personality functioning and the individual's personality trait expression are <u>not better understood as normal for an individual's developmental stage or sociocultural environment</u>.	AVPD OCPD NPD BPD ASPD STPD PD-TS

*Mark whether each of the Criteria C–G applies for any provisional personality disorder for which Criteria A and B have been met. Omit scoring if Criteria A and B have *not* been met.
Note. ASPD = Antisocial Personality Disorder; AVPD = Avoidant Personality Disorder; BPD = Borderline Personality Disorder; NPD = Narcissistic Personality Disorder; OCPD = Obsessive-Compulsive Personality Disorder; PD = Personality Disorder; PD-TS = Personality Disorder–Trait Specified (*evaluated in Part II*); STPD= Schizotypal Personality Disorder.

PART II: EVALUATION OF PERSONALITY DISORDER– TRAIT SPECIFIED

The evaluation of PD-TS begins with assessing whether Criterion A is met. Criterion A of PD-TS (i.e., "moderate or greater impairment in personality functioning, manifested by difficulties in two or more of the following four areas: 1) Identity, 2) Self-Direction, 3) Empathy, and 4) Intimacy") has been operationalized as requiring **at least one item rated "2" for at least two different domains of personality functioning.**

Summary of Criterion A (Personality Functioning) Ratings

1. IDENTITY	Rating		
AVPD A1 (page 7)	0	1	2
OCPD A1 (page 13)	0	1	2
NPD A1 (page 18)	0	1	2
BPD A1 (page 23)	0	1	2
ASPD A1 (page 33)	0	1	2
STPD A1 (page 40)	0	1	2
At least ONE is rated "2."	NO	YES	
2. SELF-DIRECTION	Rating		
AVPD A2 (page 7)	0	1	2
OCPD A2 (page 13)	0	1	2
NPD A2 (page 18)	0	1	2
BPD A2 (page 23)	0	1	2
ASPD A2 (page 33)	0	1	2
STPD A2 (page 40)	0	1	2
At least ONE is rated "2."	NO	YES	
3. EMPATHY	Rating		
AVPD A3 (page 8)	0	1	2
OCPD A3 (page 14)	0	1	2
NPD A3 (page 19)	0	1	2
BPD A3 (page 24)	0	1	2
ASPD A3 (page 34)	0	1	2
STPD A3 (page 41)	0	1	2
At least ONE is rated "2."	NO	YES	
4. INTIMACY	Rating		
AVPD A4 (page 8)	0	1	2
OCPD A4 (page 14)	0	1	2
NPD A4 (page 20)	0	1	2
BPD A4 (page 24)	0	1	2
ASPD A4 (page 34)	0	1	2
STPD A4 (page 41)	0	1	2
At least ONE is rated "2."	NO	YES	
At least __TWO__ DOMAINS are rated "YES."	NO	YES	

PD-TS Criterion A is met.

Summary of Criterion B (Personality Trait) Ratings

After assessing whether Criterion A of PD-TS is met, next assess for the presence of Criterion B. Criterion B of PD-TS ("one or more pathological personality trait domains or specific trait facets within domains") has been operationalized as **at least one trait facet rated "2" or "3."**

Note: Page numbers refer to those pages where the rating is recorded.

<table>
<tr>
<td rowspan="7" style="writing-mode: vertical-rl;">Negative Affectivity</td>
<td>Emotional Lability
Included in Borderline PD (Criterion B1), page 26</td>
<td>?   0   1   2   3</td>
</tr>
<tr>
<td>Anxiousness
Included in Avoidant PD (Criterion B1), page 9, and
in Borderline PD (Criterion B2) (separate ratings)</td>
<td>AVOIDANT PD:
?   0   1   2   3

BORDERLINE PD:
?   0   1   2   3</td>
</tr>
<tr>
<td>Separation Insecurity
Included in Borderline PD (Criterion B3), page 27</td>
<td>?   0   1   2   3</td>
</tr>
<tr>
<td>Submissiveness
Not included in any specific PD, page 46</td>
<td>?   0   1   2   3</td>
</tr>
<tr>
<td>Hostility (also an aspect of Antagonism):
Included in Borderline PD (Criterion B7), page 31, and
Antisocial PD (Criterion B4) (separate ratings)</td>
<td>BORDERLINE PD:
?   0   1   2   3

ANTISOCIAL PD:
?   0   1   2   3</td>
</tr>
<tr>
<td>Perseveration
Included in OCPD (Criterion B2), page 16</td>
<td>?   0   1   2   3</td>
</tr>
<tr>
<td colspan="2"></td>
</tr>
<tr>
<td rowspan="7" style="writing-mode: vertical-rl;">Detachment</td>
<td>Withdrawal
Included in Avoidant PD (Criterion B2), page 10, and
Schizotypal PD (Criterion B5) (separate ratings)</td>
<td>AVOIDANT PD:
?   0   1   2   3

SCHIZOTYPAL PD:
?   0   1   2   3</td>
</tr>
<tr>
<td>Intimacy Avoidance
Included in Avoidant PD (Criterion B4), page 11, and OCPD
(Criterion B3) (same rating)</td>
<td>?   0   1   2   3</td>
</tr>
<tr>
<td>Anhedonia
Included in Avoidant PD (Criterion B3), page 11</td>
<td>?   0   1   2   3</td>
</tr>
<tr>
<td>Depressivity (also an aspect of Negative Affectivity)
Included in Borderline PD (Criterion B4), page 27</td>
<td>?   0   1   2   3</td>
</tr>
<tr>
<td>Restricted Affectivity
Included in OCPD (Criterion B4), page 16, and Schizotypal PD
(Criterion B4) (same rating)</td>
<td>?   0   1   2   3</td>
</tr>
<tr>
<td>Suspiciousness (also an aspect of Negative Affectivity)
Included in Schizotypal PD (Criterion B6), page 45</td>
<td>?   0   1   2   3</td>
</tr>
</table>

(continued on next page)

Antagonism	**Manipulativeness** Included in Antisocial PD (Criterion B1), page 35	?	0	1	2	3
	Deceitfulness Included in Antisocial PD (Criterion B3), page 37	?	0	1	2	3
	Grandiosity Included in Narcissistic PD (Criterion B1), page 21	?	0	1	2	3
	Attention Seeking Included in Narcissistic PD (Criterion B2), page 22	?	0	1	2	3
	Callousness Included in Antisocial PD (Criterion B2), page 36	?	0	1	2	3
Disinhibition	**Irresponsibility** Included in Antisocial PD (Criterion B7), page 38	?	0	1	2	3
	Impulsivity Included in Borderline PD (Criterion B5), page 29, and Antisocial PD (Criterion B6) (separate ratings)	**BORDERLINE PD:** ?　0　1　2　3 **ANTISOCIAL PD:** ?　0　1　2　3				
	Distractibility Not included in any specific PD, page 46	?	0	1	2	3
	Risk Taking Included in Borderline PD (Criterion B6), page 30, and Antisocial PD (Criterion B5) (separate ratings)	**BORDERLINE PD:** ?　0　1　2　3 **ANTISOCIAL PD:** ?　0　1　2　3				
	Rigid Perfectionism (an aspect of extreme Conscientiousness, the opposite pole of Disinhibition) Included in OCPD (Criterion B1), page 15	?	0	1	2	3
Psychoticism	**Unusual Beliefs and Experiences** Included in Schizotypal PD (Criterion B2), page 43	?	0	1	2	3
	Eccentricity Included in Schizotypal (Criterion B3), page 44	?	0	1	2	3
	Cognitive and Perceptual Dysregulation Included in Schizotypal PD (Criterion B1), page 42	?	0	1	2	3
	At least ONE TRAIT FACET is rated "2" or "3."	NO		YES		

PD-TS Criterion B is met.

PD-TS CRITERION A and B are met.	NO	YES

Personality Disorder–Trait-Specified (provisional)

ONLY IF PREVIOUS ITEM RATED "YES": **ALL** of the GENERAL CRITERIA C–G ARE MET (see pages 48–49).	NO	YES

Personality Disorder–Trait-Specified (PD-TS)

PART III: RATING SEVERITY OF THE PERSONALITY DISORDER: LEVEL OF PERSONALITY FUNCTIONING SCALE

Instructions

Personality functioning is distributed across a continuum. Central to functioning and adaptation are individuals' characteristic ways of thinking about and understanding themselves and their interactions with other people. An optimally functioning person has a complex, fully elaborated, and well-integrated psychological world that includes a mostly positive, volitional, and effective self-concept; a rich, broad, and appropriately regulated emotional life; and the capacity to behave as a well-related, productive member of a society.

The Level of Personality Functioning Scale (LPFS) is comprised of the following four domains:

Self Functioning

Identity (a component of self functioning): Experience of oneself as unique, with clear boundaries between self and others; stability of self-esteem and accuracy of self-appraisal; capacity for, and ability to regulate, a range of emotional experience

Self-Direction (a component of self functioning): Pursuit of coherent and meaningful short-term and life goals; utilization of constructive and prosocial internal standards of behavior; ability to self-reflect productively

Interpersonal Functioning

Empathy (a component of interpersonal functioning): Comprehension and appreciation of others' experiences and motivations; tolerance of differing perspectives; understanding of the effects of own behavior on others

Intimacy (a component of interpersonal functioning): Depth and duration of positive connections with others; desire and capacity for closeness; mutuality of regard reflected in interpersonal behavior

Consider the complete Level of Personality Functioning Scale provided on the following pages and provide a global score between 0 and 4, using your clinical judgment based on information from the General Overview, the Preliminary Questions, and the Module III interview for Part I and Part II (the latter, if applicable).

　　　　GLOBAL SCORE: _____

Level of Personality Functioning Scale

Level of Impairment	SELF		INTERPERSONAL	
	Identity	Self-Direction	Empathy	Intimacy
0—Little or no impairment	Has ongoing awareness of a unique self; maintains role-appropriate boundaries.	Sets and aspires to reasonable goals based on a realistic assessment of personal capacities.	Is capable of accurately understanding others' experiences and motivations in most situations.	Maintains multiple satisfying and enduring relationships in personal and community life.
	Has consistent and self-regulated positive self-esteem, with accurate self-appraisal.	Utilizes appropriate standards of behavior, attaining fulfillment in multiple realms.	Comprehends and appreciates others' perspectives, even if disagreeing.	Desires and engages in a number of caring, close, and reciprocal relationships.
	Is capable of experiencing, tolerating, and regulating a full range of emotions.	Can reflect on, and make constructive meaning of, internal experience.	Is aware of the effect of own actions on others.	Strives for cooperation and mutual benefit and flexibly responds to a range of others' ideas, emotions, and behaviors.
1—Some impairment	Has relatively intact sense of self, with some decrease in clarity of boundaries when strong emotions and mental distress are experienced.	Is excessively goal-directed, somewhat goal-inhibited, or conflicted about goals.	Is somewhat compromised in ability to appreciate and understand others' experiences; may tend to see others as having unreasonable expectations or a wish for control.	Is able to establish enduring relationships in personal and community life, with some limitations on degree of depth and satisfaction.
	Self-esteem diminished at times, with overly critical or somewhat distorted self-appraisal.	May have an unrealistic or socially inappropriate set of personal standards, limiting some aspects of fulfillment.	Although capable of considering and understanding different perspectives, resists doing so.	Is capable of forming and desires to form intimate and reciprocal relationships, but may be inhibited in meaningful expression and sometimes constrained if intense emotions or conflicts arise.
	Strong emotions may be distressing, associated with a restriction in range of emotional experience.	Is able to reflect on internal experiences, but may overemphasize a single (e.g., intellectual, emotional) type of self-knowledge.	Has inconsistent awareness of effect of own behavior on others.	Cooperation may be inhibited by unrealistic standards; somewhat limited in ability to respect or respond to others' ideas, emotions, and behaviors.

Level of Personality Functioning Scale (*continued*)

| Level of Impairment | SELF | | INTERPERSONAL | |
	Identity	Self-Direction	Empathy	Intimacy
2—Moderate impairment	Depends excessively on others for identity definition, with compromised boundary delineation. Has vulnerable self-esteem controlled by exaggerated concern about external evaluation, with a wish for approval. Has sense of incompleteness or inferiority, with compensatory inflated, or deflated, self-appraisal. Emotional regulation depends on positive external appraisal. Threats to self-esteem may engender strong emotions such as rage or shame.	Goals are more often a means of gaining external approval than self-generated, and thus may lack coherence and/or stability. Personal standards may be unreasonably high (e.g., a need to be special or please others) or low (e.g., not consonant with prevailing social values). Fulfillment is compromised by a sense of lack of authenticity. Has impaired capacity to reflect on internal experience.	Is hyperattuned to the experience of others, but only with respect to perceived relevance to self. Is excessively self-referential; significantly compromised ability to appreciate and understand others' experiences and to consider alternative perspectives. Is generally unaware of or unconcerned about effect of own behavior on others, or unrealistic appraisal of own effect.	Is capable of forming and desires to form relationships in personal and community life, but connections may be largely superficial. Intimate relationships are predominantly based on meeting self-regulatory and self-esteem needs, with an unrealistic expectation of being perfectly understood by others. Tends not to view relationships in reciprocal terms, and cooperates predominantly for personal gain.

Level of Personality Functioning Scale (*continued*)

Level of Impairment	SELF		INTERPERSONAL	
	Identity	Self-Direction	Empathy	Intimacy
3—Severe impairment	Has a weak sense of autonomy/agency; experience of a lack of identity, or emptiness. Boundary definition is poor or rigid: may show overidentification with others, overemphasis on independence from others, or vacillation between these. Fragile self-esteem is easily influenced by events, and self-image lacks coherence. Self-appraisal is un-nuanced: self-loathing, self-aggrandizing, or an illogical, unrealistic combination. Emotions may be rapidly shifting or a chronic, unwavering feeling of despair.	Has difficulty establishing and/or achieving personal goals. Internal standards for behavior are unclear or contradictory. Life is experienced as meaningless or dangerous. Has significantly compromised ability to reflect on and understand own mental processes.	Ability to consider and understand the thoughts, feelings, and behavior of other people is significantly limited; may discern very specific aspects of others' experience, particularly vulnerabilities and suffering. Is generally unable to consider alternative perspectives; highly threatened by differences of opinion or alternative viewpoints. Is confused about or unaware of impact of own actions on others; often bewildered about people's thoughts and actions, with destructive motivations frequently misattributed to others.	Has some desire to form relationships in community and personal life, but capacity for positive and enduring connections is significantly impaired. Relationships are based on a strong belief in the absolute need for the intimate other(s), and/or expectations of abandonment or abuse. Feelings about intimate involvement with others alternate between fear/rejection and desperate desire for connection. Little mutuality: others are conceptualized primarily in terms of how they affect the self (negatively or positively); cooperative efforts are often disrupted due to the perception of slights from others.

Level of Personality Functioning Scale (continued)

Level of Impairment	SELF		INTERPERSONAL	
	Identity	**Self-Direction**	**Empathy**	**Intimacy**
4—Extreme impairment	Experience of a unique self and sense of agency/autonomy are virtually absent, or are organized around perceived external persecution. Boundaries with others are confused or lacking.	Has poor differentiation of thoughts from actions, so goal-setting ability is severely compromised, with unrealistic or incoherent goals.	Has pronounced inability to consider and understand others' experience and motivation.	Desire for affiliation is limited because of profound disinterest or expectation of harm. Engagement with others is detached, disorganized, or consistently negative.
	Has weak or distorted self-image easily threatened by interactions with others; significant distortions and confusion around self-appraisal.	Internal standards for behavior are virtually lacking. Genuine fulfillment is virtually inconceivable.	Attention to others' perspectives is virtually absent (attention is hypervigilant, focused on need fulfillment and harm avoidance).	Relationships are conceptualized almost exclusively in terms of their ability to provide comfort or inflict pain and suffering.
	Emotions not congruent with context or internal experience. Hatred and aggression may be dominant affects, although they may be disavowed and attributed to others.	Is profoundly unable to constructively reflect on own experience. Personal motivations may be unrecognized and/or experienced as external to self.	Social interactions can be confusing and disorienting.	Social/interpersonal behavior is not reciprocal; rather, it seeks fulfillment of basic needs or escape from pain.

EXPERTLY DESIGNED, the *Structured Clinical Interview for the DSM-5® Alternative Model for Personality Disorders* (SCID-5-AMPD) is a semi-structured diagnostic interview that guides clear assessment of the defining components of personality pathology as presented in the DSM-5 Alternative Model. The modular format of the SCID-5-AMPD allows the researcher or clinician to focus on those aspects of the Alternative Model of most interest.

Module III: Structured Clinical Interview for Personality Disorders (Including Personality Disorder–Trait Specified) provides a comprehensive assessment of each of the six specific personality disorders of the Alternative Model (Antisocial Personality Disorder, Avoidant Personality Disorder, Borderline Personality Disorder, Narcissistic Personality Disorder, Obsessive-Compulsive Personality Disorder, and Schizotypal Personality Disorder) as well as Personality Disorder–Trait Specified, which can be diagnosed if criteria are not met for any of the six specific disorders. The module concludes with a global assessment of the level of personality functioning and includes a summary of all the personality disorder diagnoses in the module.

Module III can be used independently or in combination with any of the following SCID-5-AMPD modules:

- **Module I** dimensionally assesses self and interpersonal functioning using the Level of Personality Functioning Scale.

- **Module II** dimensionally assesses the five pathological personality trait domains and their corresponding 25 trait facets.

Also available is the **User's Guide for the SCID-5-AMPD:** the essential tool for the effective use of each SCID-5-AMPD module. This companion guide provides instructions for each SCID-5-AMPD module and features completed samples of all modules in full, with corresponding sample patient cases and commentary.

Trained clinicians with a basic knowledge of the concepts of personality and personality psychopathology will benefit from the myriad applications and perspectives offered by the SCID-5-AMPD.

MICHAEL B. FIRST, M.D., is Professor of Clinical Psychiatry at Columbia University College of Physicians and Surgeons, and Research Psychiatrist in the Division of Clinical Phenomenology at the New York State Psychiatric Institute in New York, New York.

ANDREW E. SKODOL, M.D., is Research Professor of Psychiatry at the University of Arizona College of Medicine in Tucson, Arizona, and Adjunct Professor of Psychiatry at Columbia University College of Physicians and Surgeons in New York, New York.

DONNA S. BENDER, PH.D., is Director, Counseling and Psychological Services, and Clinical Professor of Psychiatry and Behavioral Sciences at Tulane University in New Orleans, Louisiana.

JOHN M. OLDHAM, M.D., is Professor of Psychiatry and Barbara and Corbin Robertson Jr. Endowed Chair for Personality Disorders at Baylor College of Medicine in Houston, Texas.

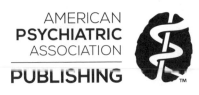

AMERICAN
PSYCHIATRIC
ASSOCIATION
PUBLISHING

WWW.APPI.ORG